The amazing
Liver and Gallbladder Flush

–

A Step-by-Step Guide
based on Andreas Moritz Miracle Cleanse

Your All-Natural, At-Home Liver Detox, Cleanse & Repair
to Purify and Rejuvenate Your Body
with Timeless Secrets of Health and Rejuvenation

Table of contents

Foreword

Andreas Moritz's original bestselling book is entitled "The Amazing Liver and Gallbladder Flush" and has sold over 1 million copies worldwide. The book has almost 500 pages and teaches the willing reader all the detailed knowledge about the liver and gallbladder.

The actual steps of the flush itself are then not explained very clearly, hidden between pages 293 and 297. There is no shopping list, there are no clear illustrations of the cleansing process, there is no timetable and so on. The book by Andreas Moritz can therefore hardly be used as a practical guide to carrying out a liver and gallbladder cleanse.

Therefore, as huge proponents of the liver and gallbladder cleanse (also called liver flush), we have created a step-by-step guide with this book. We have summarized the relevant knowledge from Andreas Moritz' book and presented it clearly. We go into all the important topics related to the cleanse. In this book you will not be trained to become a health expert, but you will receive all the relevant practical instructions!

Much success!

1 Liver and Gallbladder Flush 101

The cleansing is carried out regularly by many fans and is considered by them to be one of the most important and effective methods to improve their own health.

Part of this cleansing method involves a brief fasting period, which in itself yields plentiful positive health effects. These benefits alone could make the liver and gallbladder flush come highly recommended.

We acknowledge that Andreas Moritz's method boasts both fervent supporters and staunch critics. With that in mind, we will briefly delve into potential risks, ensuring that this summary equips you with a well-rounded understanding.

The method

The cleansing stimulates the production of bile in the gallbladder. As a result of this method, a particularly large amount of bile is produced and consequently it is discharged from the body through the digestive tract. This process is cleansing and, according to Andreas Moritz, should also loosen and drain old gallstones.

The cleanse is comprised of a 6-day preparation period followed by the cleansing phase, with brief fasting bridging the gap between these two stages.

Preparation phase (6 days)**:**
Throughout the six-day preparation phase, a substantial amount of juice is consumed to facilitate the gentle dissolution of gallstones.

Furthermore, it's important to adhere to specific dietary guidelines during this preparation period, which we will discuss shortly.

Cleansing phase (20 hours)**:**
Following the six-day preparation phase, the actual cleansing process starts and typically spans around 20 hours.

The cleansing procedure begins with the consumption of a blend of olive oil and grapefruit. Throughout this period, it's advised to remain in proximity to a toilet at all times (though this might sound more daunting than it truly is).

Hence, the weekend is particularly convenient for undertaking the cleansing phase. Starting with the preparation phase on a Monday will enable you to use the weekend for the cleanse.

2 The Risks

As mentioned, we also want to briefly touch on the risks of a liver and gallbladder cleanse.

If you suffer from one of the following diseases or belong to one of the risk groups listed, you should <u>not</u> carry out the cleansing.

2.1 Gallstones

Individuals suffering from gallstones are frequently cautioned against self-administering the Andreas Moritz method for treatment.

This caution stems from the fact that the gallbladder experiences significant contractions during the cleansing process in order to expel bile. This contraction can potentially trigger colic in individuals suffering from gallstones.

Andreas Moritz himself says that the existing gallstones were significantly softened during the six-day preparation phase. According to him, this softening diminishes any impediments to his treatment approach.

2.2 Constipation

If you experience mild constipation, it's recommended to perform a self-administered enema both after the preparation period and before entering the cleansing phase.

The enema assists the body in effectively expelling the toxins generated by the gallbladder cleansing process. This ensures that these toxins are not reabsorbed due to constipation within the body.

2.3 Risk Groups

A liver and gallbladder cleanse should <u>not</u> be performed by people:

- In chemotherapy treatment / with cancer
- With stents in the bile duct (artificial tube)
- With diabetes
- With intestinal obstructions / hemorrhoids
- With acute infections or medication prescribed by a doctor
- With bloody stool
- With hypoglycemia
- With yeast infection (e.g. candida)
- With stomach ulcers

Additionally, please take note: Women who are currently menstruating, pregnant, or breastfeeding should avoid undergoing a liver and gallbladder flush during this period.

3 Essential Supplies for the Flush

Within this chapter, our aim is to outline the essential foods crucial for a liver and gallbladder flush. Furthermore, we will provide concise explanations detailing the reasons and mechanisms through which each food item contributes to your cleansing process.

3.1 Juice for preparation phase

In the period of preparation, you need to drink juice every day. Take apple or tart cherry juice (sometimes called sour cherry juice).

The malic acid found in apple juice or tart cherry juice has a softening effect on gallstones, allowing them to pass through the ducts smoothly.

According to Andreas Moritz, apple juice and tart cherry juice are equally suitable for preparing the liver and gallbladder for an effective flush. However, pay attention to the different quantities described below!

Also, make sure the juices are organic and don't contain any food preservatives.

3.1.1 Apple juice (32 oz. per day)

If you want to use apple juice for the preparation phase, it is best to use organic juice. Freshly prepared juice from organic apples is particularly recommended. Drink 32 oz. per day of preparation!

Both clear apple juice and naturally cloudy apple juice or concentrate are suitable. To prevent the malic acid it contains from affecting your teeth, it's advisable to thoroughly rinse your mouth or brush your teeth after consumption.

3.1.2   Tart cherry juice (8 oz. per day)

Caution: tart / sour cherries should not be confused with sweet cherries.

The content of malic acid in tart cherries is about four times higher than that in apples. Therefore, when choosing tart cherry juice, you only need a quarter of the amount compared to apple juice.

Be sure to buy unsweetened tart cherry juice in glass bottles!

3.2 Dietary guidelines for the preparation phase

Drink a lot of water! Andreas Moritz emphasizes again and again: in order for the body to be able to produce enough bile, it needs a particularly large amount of water. A lot of water is also important and necessary for flushing out the stones from the liver and bile.

In addition, adhere to the following nutritional guidelines during the preparation phase:

Dietary guidelines during preparation phase
- No ice-cold food/drinks, as these have a liver-straining effect
- No food of animal origin (meat, fish, eggs, milk... but butter is ok)
- No refined sugar (honey is a good alternative)
- No fried foods

3.3 Grapefruit and olive oil for the cleansing phase

3.3.1 Grapefruits
Purchase 2-3 grapefruits, each at least the size of your fist. When buying the grapefruits, it's vital to prioritize those that are "organic," given that they will be used for squeezing. This precaution is essential to prevent the potential extraction of chemicals which may have been applied to the peel during cultivation.

3.3.2 Extra Virgin Olive Oil

For the cleanse it is vital that you use the highest quality of olive oil. This is the extra virgin olive oil - also known as "olio d'olivia extra virgin". Exercise diligence in inspecting the label thoroughly. Specifically, ensure that it doesn't include ingredients like soybean oil or other oils that are deemed subpar for this particular purpose. Definitely stay clear of refined vegetable / seed oils.

Avoid buying olive oil packaged in plastic bottles! Similar to premium red wine or high-quality beer, you can distinguish excellent olive oil in part by its packaging — often presented in darkened glass bottles.

3.3.3 Clean sealable glass jar

Because the squeezed grapefruit juice is mixed with the olive oil by shaking, it's necessary to have an empty, sealable jar for this purpose.

Cleaned jam jars are a good option for this. Alternatively, a cocktail shaker will also do the job.

3.4 Summary: Shopping List

- Apple juice   6x 32 oz. containers
  = 6 liters

  or
  Tart / sour cherry juice   6x 8 oz. portions
  = 1.5 liters

- Extra Virgin Olive Oil   4 oz. / ½ cup / 120ml

- Grapefruit juice   6 oz. / ¾ cup / 180ml
  = 2-3 large grapefruits

- Epsom salt*   4 tablespoons / ¼ cup
  = 5-6 epsom capsules

- Lemon squeezer to extract grapefruit juice from the fruit

- Empty sealable jam jar with a minimum volume of at least 10 oz (used as shaker).

*) Epsom salt is also know as magnesium sulfate or magnesium citrate

4 The Cleansing

The preparation phase spans 6 days. You'll follow a vegetarian diet and drink your juice daily. Throughout this period, you can continue your regular work and don't need to focus on anything else.

The cleansing phase starts on the 6th day and ends on the 7th day. Therefore, many people start the preparation phase of the flush on Monday and finish the cleanse on Sunday.

As an option, a colon hydrotherapy session can be booked for the subsequent Monday.

4.1 Preparation Phase (Day 1 – 6)

Consume your juice daily during the initial six days, either in its pure form or diluted by adding water to the original amount.

The significantly increased juice intake possesses a potent cleansing effect. In individuals with heightened sensitivity, this abundance of juice might potentially result in a sense of fullness or even diarrhea. The diarrhea might indeed indicate the release of bile that was previously stored in the liver and gallbladder, identifiable by its brownish/yellowish color. However, it's important to note that diarrhea could also stem from the fermentation of sugar present in the juice.

Consume the juice slowly and in small portions throughout the day, making sure to have it exclusively between meals.

Nonetheless, it's advisable not to consume juice right before a meal, within the initial one to two hours after a meal, and in the evening after 6 p.m. In every circumstance, the juice should be ingested alongside the regular daily water intake of 6 to 8 glasses.

Note: On the sixth day of the preparation period, consume the entire quantity of juice in the morning.

Kindly adhere rigorously to the specified dietary guidelines.

4.2 The 6th day of the preparation period

Consume the daily quantity of apple juice or tart cherry juice in the morning, preferably right after waking up. Opt for a light breakfast, like fruit or a warm oatmeal.

Avoid sugar and sweeteners, spices, milk, butter, oil, yogurt, cheese, ham, eggs, nuts, pastries, cold cereals, and other processed foods. Conversely, freshly prepared fruit or vegetable juices are permissible.

For lunch, opt for lightly boiled or steamed vegetables served with rice (white basmati rice is recommended), buckwheat, quinoa, or a similar option. Flavor the meal with a touch of unrefined sea or rock salt.

Alternatively, you can choose raw fruits or vegetables if that's your preference.

Steer clear of protein and fatty foods (such as nuts, avocados, butter, or oil) as they may lead to discomfort during the actual cleansing phase. It's crucial to conserve as much bile as possible for the liver flush. This bile is essential to effectively expel a substantial number of stones from the liver and gallbladder. Consuming fatty foods would prompt the body to utilize this bile for digestion, compromising the cleansing process.

The preparation phase ends with lunch on the sixth day.

4.3 The cleansing phase (day 6 and 7)

Abstain from eating during the cleansing phase. Consume only water throughout the entire afternoon of day 6, preferably in ample quantities, as the body will require it for the forthcoming evening bile flush.

On the evening of the sixth day (starting at 6:00 p.m.), initiate the consumption of the cleansing substances.

6:00 p.m.:

Use a teapot or glass carafe to dissolve 4 tablespoons of epsom salts in 24 oz. / 3 cups / 700ml of water (filtered is best). Divide the mixture into four glasses. This gives you four portions of 6 oz. / 175 ml each. Drink the first portion now.

Andreas Moritz identifies the relaxation and widening of the bile ducts as the most important task of epsom salt. This should make it easier for the stones to be flushed out.

If you find the bitter taste challenging, you can easily mitigate it by adding a bit of lemon juice. Another option is to rinse your mouth with water after consumption. If the mixture remains challenging to drink, you can use a straw to bypass the taste buds on your tongue. Holding your nose while drinking can help suppress the taste as well.

8:00 p.m.:
<u>Drink </u>the second serving of Epsom salts.

9:30 p.m.:
If the Epsom salts haven't yet prompted a bowel movement, you can opt to use an enema to stimulate one. But if you've been sticking to the plan so far, you've probably had to go to the bathroom by now.

Caution: Please make sure that you only continue the flushing if you have had a bowel movement in this step. Avoiding constipation is of paramount importance.

9:45 p.m.:
Squeeze the grapefruits after washing them thoroughly. The juice is required without the pulp - a total of 6 oz. / ¾ cup / 180ml.

Now mix the 6 oz. of grapefruit juice with the 4 oz. / ½ cup / 120ml of olive oil. A washed-out jam jar, for example, is ideal for this. Now shake the mixture vigorously so that the oil and juice will blend.

10:00 p.m.:

Give the mixture another good shake and consume it all in a single gulp. Subsequently, head straight to bed. If needed, you can brush your teeth beforehand, although it's advised to go to bed promptly after ingesting the mixture.

Starting now, refrain from drinking any water for a minimum of 2 hours. Now, **IMMEDIATELY LIE DOWN AND REMAIN MOTIONLESS FOR AT LEAST 20 MINUTES**. Turn off the lights and avoid speaking as well. This step is highly crucial to aid in dissolving the gallstones. Be certain that your head is positioned notably higher than your stomach. If needed, use multiple pillows to achieve this elevation. Failing to do so might lead to nausea.

Alternatively, if lying on your back is exceptionally uncomfortable, lie on your right side and pull your knees toward your stomach.

Once the initial 20 minutes have passed, you can resume your regular sleeping position. However, be sure to avoid lying on your stomach.

The next morning (Day 7)

6:00 a.m.:
Drink a glass of warm water.

6:15 a.m.:
Drink the third serving of Epsom salts. If you prefer not to go back to sleep, you can engage in reading or meditation. Maintaining an upright body position is recommended. Refrain from consuming water for up to 15 minutes after ingesting Epsom salts.

8:15 a.m.:
Drink the fourth and final serving of Epsom salts.

Once you visit the bathroom, you may notice small green globules in your stool. Andreas Moritz suggests that these are the gallstones that have been loosened. Critics argue that these might be the saponified remnants of oil and Epsom salts. Regardless of the viewpoint, you'll likely experience a sensation of increased lightness and clarity following the liver flush.

From 10:30 a.m.:
At this point, you can enjoy a freshly squeezed fruit juice and indulge in a few pieces of fruit after some time has passed.

From 12:00 p.m.: 2 options

Option 1: You can now resume your regular eating habits. It's beneficial to opt for a light and vegetarian meal at this stage, ensuring you stop eating before you feel overly full.

Option 2: Alternatively, you can continue fasting, drink plenty of water, and consume only a few pieces of fruit. The same evening or the following day, consider undergoing a colon hydrotherapy session to expel the toxins resulting from the cleansing process from your colon. This procedure also aids in flushing out the yellowish bile produced during the cleansing, which accumulates in the intestines.

The Step-by-Step Guide for the Liver and Gallbladder Flush

according to Andreas Moritz:

5 Step-by-step guide

Preparation phase (5 days)
- Stick to dietary requirements
- Drink the amount of juice every day until 6 p.m. (not around meals)

Preparation phase (6th day in the morning)
- Eat only a light breakfast and stick to dietary guidelines
- Drink the amount of juice by 12 p.m. (not around meals)
- Midday small lunch e.g. raw or steamed vegetables with rice/ quinoa; alternatively raw fruit / vegetables (avoid protein and fats in any case!)
- Fast from 1:30 p.m. and only drink a lot of water

Cleansing day (6th day in the afternoon)
- Afternoon: No food, just drink plenty of water
- 6:00 p.m.:   1st portion of Epsom salt + 15min no water
- 8:00 p.m.:   2nd portion of Epsom salt + 15min no water
- 9:30 p.m.:   enema if necessary to trigger bowel movements
- 9:45 p.m.:   Prepare the grapefruit oil mixture
- 10:00 p.m.:   Drink the grapefruit oil mixture
- Afterwards: straight to bed, head elevated, motionless for 20 minutes
- Sleeping: Sleep on your back or right side

Recovery day (7th day)

- 6:00 a.m.:   Drink 1 glass of warm water
- 6:15 a.m.: 3rd portion of Epsom salt + 15min no water
- 8:15 a.m.: 4th portion of Epsom salt +15min no water
- 10:30 a.m.:   Freshly squeezed fruit juice
- 11:00 a.m.:   One or two pieces of fruit
- From 12 p.m.: Eat normally again (light, vegetarian) or

  Optional: Continue fasting for colon hydrotherapy in the evening of day 7 or on day 8

Optional: colon hydrotherapy (7th or 8th day)

The flush triggers the body to expel accumulated toxins. To prevent these toxins from lingering in the intestines and potentially being reabsorbed, it's **highly advisable** to undergo an intestinal cleansing on the evening of the 7th day or the 8th day.

More precisely, it is recommended to opt for a professionally administered colon hydrotherapy, which typically includes a stomach massage. This procedure, costing around $100 - $150, effectively flushes your bowels with water, promoting a cleansing effect. It's common to observe the expulsion of remnants of the distinct yellowish bile during this process.

Particularly knowledgeable providers administer probiotics as part of the colon hydrotherapy, aiding in the restoration of your gut flora and fostering a healthy balance of intestinal bacteria. Especially after a cleansing process, the effectiveness of a probiotics treatment is notably enhanced.

You're very welcome for exploring this step-by-step guide. We trust it has proven valuable for your cleanse and would greatly appreciate your review. The positive effects of this cleanse will likely resonate with you for an extended period, particularly if you chose to undergo colon hydrotherapy.

Made in the USA
Thornton, CO
01/05/25 21:51:36